1

HOW I DEFEATED MENOPAUSAL HOT FLUSHES

Dr. C. Brusi hMD
Internal Medicine Consultant

Index

Introduction	page 6
What menopause is	page 9
Symptoms and complications	page 14
Hot flushes	page 17
Useful tips	page 21
The importance of nutrition	page 28
Other natural remedies	page 30
Pharmacological therapy	page 38
How I solved the problem of hot flushes	page 42
Conclusion	page 65

Bibliography   page 67

Introduction

This booklet does not pretend to be a scientific text containing effective and tested therapies to counter the signs and symptoms of the menopause, but to provide the basis for a deeper knowledge of this natural phase of change in a woman's life, some practical advice, some natural remedies and my personal method, an effective result, to defeat the most known, hated and feared disorder: hot flushes.

The content of these pages is intended for informational purposes only, and under no circumstances should be used as a substitute for the formulation of a diagnosis or the prescription of a treatment. Also, it should not replace the doctor-patient relationship. I therefore recommend all readers to always contact their doctor and/or trusted specialists before putting into practice the advice and suggestions indicated. If you have any doubt, contact your doctor before taking any medicinal product.

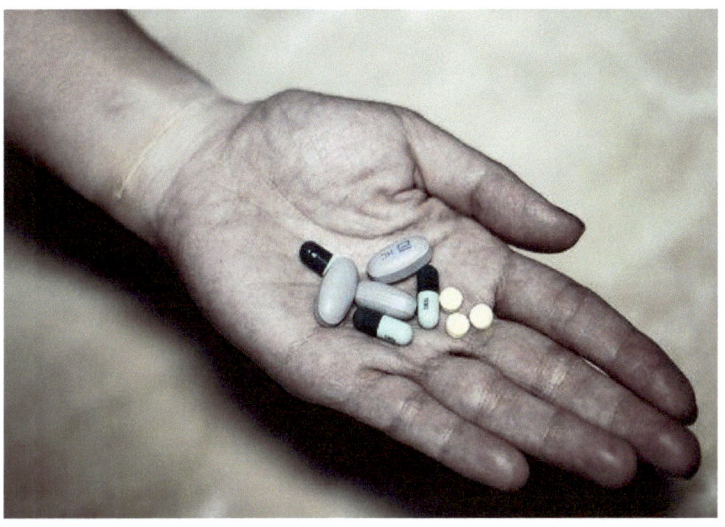

What menopause is

The menopause is a "complex and still largely unknown set of genetic, hormonal and environmental factors (Nature)". In fact, there are several aspects that Science still cannot explain about the menopause: what it is for, how it works, and above all, what is the best way to treat it.

It is not just the end of the female cycle.

Beyond the biological phenomenon, the entrance of the woman into the menopause represents an important transition, which marks the end of the reproductive period and the beginning of old age, with consequences of a social and psychological nature. Not only in fact, have we to confront our own physical changes, but also the changes in the image we had of our self. The menopause can also cause physical and mental discomfort, which sometimes can even compromise the woman's serenity or her relationships. To all of this are added preconceptions, beliefs and neglect, which in the past reflected a certain way of thinking about the woman's body, relegated to the mere role of procreation. Ultimately, for many years women's mental disorders and mental illnesses were widely attributed to "uterine problems", a reason why during the course of history, menopausal or post-menopausal women were considered asexual, shrewish, hysterical, dangerous, useless, and so on.

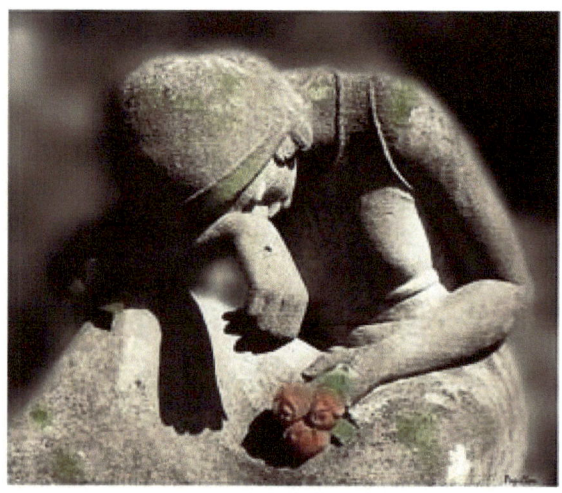

Menopause derives from the Greek words that mean "month" and "cessation" and was first used in 1821 by the French physician Charles Pierre Louis de Gardenne in the preface to his work dedicated to the critical age of women: *"De la ménopause ou de l'âge critique des femmes "*.

From the strictly medical point of view, it is the physiological phase in the life of a woman characterized by the absence of menstruation and the loss of fertility. The menopause is preceded by the "climacteric" (from the Greek klimactèr = passage/step), a transitional period of varying duration, on average lasting several years, in which a whole series of physical and psychological changes occur, following the progressive reduction in the production of hormones, progesterone and estrogen.

A recent American study published on JAMA Internal Medicine (2015), after analyzing 1500 women in the period from pre-post-menopause, has placed the duration of the climacteric between 7 and 17 years, noting that the disorders can last long time, especially those occurring during the pre-menopause. Related factors are a lower age at the first onset of sweating and flushing, a greater perception of a state of stress or anxiety, a greater sensitivity to symptoms, and a lower level of education.

The climacteric can also occur in men, in this case preceding the **Andropause** (i.e. the male menopause).

The climacteric usually occurs between 45 and 50 years of age in a woman, following the involution of the functional activity of the ovaries (the number of eggs is already established since birth and at the time of menopause all of them have disappeared) which, together with a consequent lack of estrogens circulating in the blood, cause changes in the rhythm and amount of menstrual flow. If that occurs before the age of 40-45, is called an <u>early menopause</u>, after the age of 55 we talk about <u>late menopause</u>.

The climacteric comprises of three different phases:

•**pre-menopause**: irregular menstrual cycle starts (close and abundant flows or with spaces between them) and the first symptoms, which signal the decline of the ovarian function; with the progressive reduction of hormonal levels, menstruation becomes less and less frequent, until it ceases altogether (amenorrhea).

·menopause: calculated from the twelfth consecutive month of amenorrhea after the last menstrual period; the ovaries stop producing eggs.

·post-menopause: phase in which symptoms can continue or disappear completely, generally tends to appear after 60 years of age and lasts until full senility.

The irregularities of menstrual cycle consist mainly of changes in the rhythm of the cycle (*oligomenorrhea* if the interval is more than 35 days and less than 3 months, *amenorrhea* if more than 3 months), abnormal increase in its frequency (*polymenorrhea*) and abundant loss of blood concurrent with menstruation or uterine loss between one cycle and another (*menometrorrhagia*).

Symptoms and complications

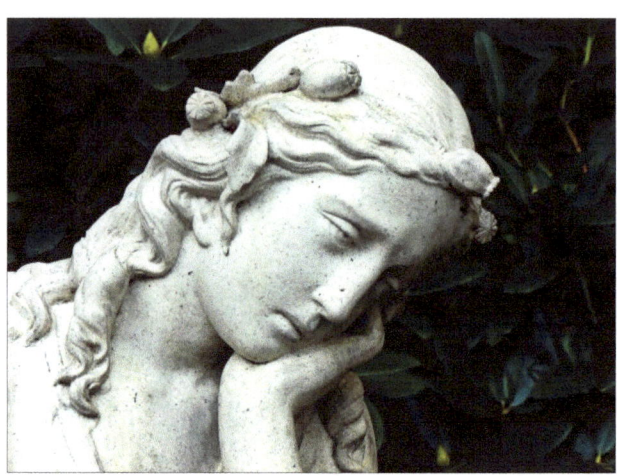

The variations in hormone levels occur to a different extent in the female population, in fact about two thirds of women face important negative effects both physically and mentally, while a third has only slight or no symptoms. Estrogens are hormones involved in various bodily functions and their receptors are found in cells throughout the body, so their deficiency determines significant consequences with symptoms and signs predominantly of a neurovegetative nature and psycho-affective disorders in the short to medium term; moreover, there are medium-long term consequences in the osteo-articular and cardio-vascular system, in genitourinary tract and on the general health conditions of women.

The most important symptoms and signs are:

- hot flushes
- night sweats
- dizziness
- transient palpitations / tachycardias
- pressure overhang
- vaginal dryness and itching
- headache
- insomnia
- increase in body weight
- mood instability, irritability, nervousness, anxiety, poor concentration and memory disturbances
- decrease in sexual desire
- cystitis and bladder trigono syndrome
- vaginitis
- dyspareunia (pain during sexual intercourse)

- depression
- incontinence or increased frequency of urinations
- hair loss and changes in skin trophism

In addition there is an increase in cardio-vascular risk and osteoarticular diseases (osteopenia, osteoporosis, joint pain).

Frequency of the main climacteric problems:

Weight gain	60%
Fatigue	43%
Profuse sweating	39%
Insomnia	32%
Hot flushes	55%
Nervousness	41%
Migraine	38%
Depression	30%

Hot flushes

They are often described as waves of sudden heat of undefined provenance, which sometimes can involve the whole body, but more often rise from the chest to the face and neck; they can be followed by profuse sweating that disappears after a few minutes, sometimes leaving the body shivering.

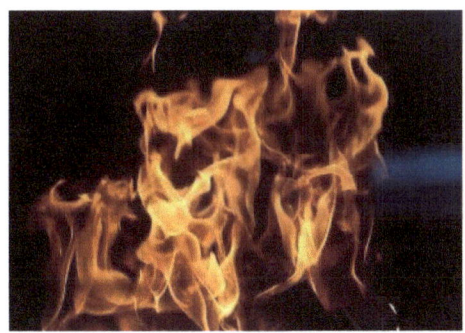

During a flush, the skin temperature rises considerably, passing within a few minutes from the usual 28-30° to 34-35° C. Hot flushes are sometimes accompanied by redness of the face, anxiety and palpitation and can appear several times during the day and night (night sweats). Some women experience occasional and light flushes, with cause little impact on their quality of life, while others can suffer 20 or more episodes a day, which can be intense and debilitating and are perceived as obstacles to everyday life. In all cases they tend to be reduced with the passage of time. On average, hot flushes affect 70% of women and they begin to appear, generally speaking, towards 47-48 years of age, together with the first major changes in the menstrual cycle. The sooner they occur, the longer they tend to recur. Hot flushes in particular, are more intense and bothersome in case of an early menopause (of natural origin or as a direct consequence of surgical removal of the ovaries or of an anticancer therapy), whilst they occur, more or less frequently, in seven out of ten women who have undergone a treatment for breast cancer. In the latter, because of the induced reduction of estrogen levels, hot flushes are often more intense than those perceived during the physiological menopause. Even men can experience hot flushes due to reduced circulating testosterone levels, as a result of prostate cancer therapy.

Some researchers have found that women suffering from hot flushes have their brain thermostat (the mechanism that regulates body temperature) much more sensitive than the average, so they are only at ease in a very small temperature range.

In fact, it seems that several areas of the brain in women with hot flushes are more susceptible to endogenous opioid deficiency secondary to hypoestrogenism, first of all the hypothalamus, the structure that regulates our whole neurovegetative life (blood pressure, body temperature, cardiac rhythm, circadian rhythm, ie sleep-wake, hormone level, etc); for this reason the hot flushes are often associated with nocturnal tachycardias, insomnia, hypertension. The profuse sweating that follows the hot flushes reflects the activation of the hypothalamus to bring the body temperature back to normal levels.

In case of persistence of the symptoms, the second area of the brain suffering is the limbic lobe, responsible for the control of mood (about a third of menopausal women suffering from hot flushes and insomnia face depression, partly because of the direct effect of estrogenic deficiency, partly due to poor quality of sleep and reduced quality of life). The third area affected is the cognitive cortex, responsible for processing the thoughts, and the first signs of the process are difficulties in remembering names, in concentrating and the tendency to lose the thread of discourse. Serious dementia may appear after ten to fifteen years, when about 80% of the nerve cells that preside over thought and memory have already been destroyed; at this point the therapies are not effective and dementia is a path with no return. Symptoms include complete loss of memory (amnesia), which begins with the inability to remember sporadic events of everyday life, then extends to "perspective" memory (keep in mind the week's commitments), to the "retrograde" memory (remembering the events of the past) and the "semantic" memory (which preserves the knowledge acquired in the course of life). Other symptoms are the difficulty to understand the words of others and to speak appropriately (aphasia), to perform actions aimed at a goal, such as taking a bottle to pour water into a glass (apraxia).

The lack of estrogens and testosterone can also affect a fourth area of the brain, the one that presides over the movement, favouring the
insurgence of Parkinson's disease, which appears when 80% of the nerve cells that co-ordinate the movements are destroyed.

Useful tips

Several precautions can be taken against hot flushes and night sweats, but first of all you have to try to change your lifestyle. Some doctors recommend insisting with these changes for at least 3 months before starting any drug therapies.

• It can be useful to dress in layers with light, thin and breathable clothes and choose sheets strictly in linen or cotton, which allows the skin to breathe better and reduce its heat.

• Keep antiperspirant wet wipes handy at all times of the day, eliminating excess sweating and preventing them from forming, leaving the skin soft and dry.

• To improve sleep, follow a regular schedule, going to bed and getting up every day at the same time; avoid, if possible, naps in the late afternoon and in the evening; develop a ritual before going to bed, such as reading, listening to music or relaxing with a hot bath; do not watch television, use computers or other mobile devices in the bedroom: their light can hinder sleep; keep a comfortable temperature in the bedroom.

• Try different strategies to stay cool during the night, for example, in place of a single blanket, use several layers that you can easily remove. Or place under the pillow a wet and frozen cloth or an ice bag in such a way that, turning the pillow, the head always stays on a cold surface. Try to drink small quantities of cold water before going to bed and keep a glass of cold water on the bedside table, in case you wake up at night.

• Try different techniques to encourage the sleep recovery in case of awakening, such as meditation or a deep, controlled rhythmic breathing.

• Keep the environment as fresh and ventilated as possible, using fans, air conditioners or a simple folding fan if necessary.

• Perform regular physical exercise, preferably aerobic, which increases the body's thermoregulatory capacities; for this reason, women who constantly perform a certain motor activity experience less intense and frequent flushes than the more sedentary women. The ideal condition would be to perform at least 30 minutes a day of gymnastics, with the precaution of interrupting at least three hours before going to sleep, to prevent night sweats. Physical activity also allows you to keep fit, improve mood, fight weight gain, protect bone mass and heart, and prevent and counter the forms of osteoarthritis associated with menopause.

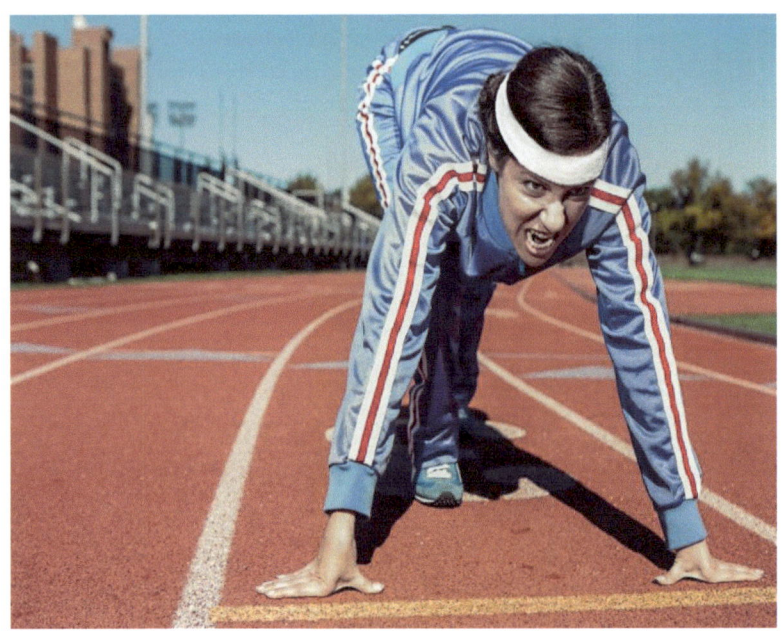

• Maintaining a normal body weight: excess of body fat provides thermal insulation that can prevent heat loss. However, it has also been shown that overweight or obese women may suffer more from frequent and severe flushes.

• Stop smoking completely: among the numerous disadvantages of smoking, it should be included its aggravating effect on the severity of the flushes, due to the accentuation of vagal activity by nicotine. Also to be linked to smoking, are greater risks of appearance of the early menopause and the insurgence of osteoporotic and cardiovascular complications.

• Keep calm and reduce the stress by practicing yoga, meditation, tai chi, qigong, biofeedback, autogenic training, acupuncture or even massages and other relaxation techniques. Avoiding triggering factors, such as bright lights or predictable emotional reactions, can also help.

• Improving breathing, for example by practicing relaxation techniques, is an effective way to reduce stress. It is basically a deep inhalation followed by an exhalation with a uniform rhythm. It should be practiced for several minutes in a comfortable position and is based on inhaling slowly from the nose. With the hand resting immediately under the ribs, in correspondence of the stomach, one must have the sensation that the latter pushes the hand away before the expansion of the thorax; then slowly exhale from the mouth, emptying firstly the lungs, and then the stomach will come back. This technique can be practiced almost anywhere and for several times during the day, whenever you feel stressed. You can also use it when you feel like you start a hot flash or relax before falling asleep. Particularly when a flush comes you must try to do 5 to 7 breaths per minute, breathing much slower than usual.

• Adopting a suitable diet. With the arrival of the menopause it becomes necessary for women to change their eating habits considering the slowing down of the metabolism and accompanying a diet with physical activity. Better avoiding very hot drinks and hot food, alcohol, caffeine, spices, spicy foods, preserved foods (as they contain substances that increase the levels of certain neurotransmitters). The food should be light and varied and low in fat content, especially in summer or in the evening. It is also important to limit the consumption of salt, sugars and refined carbohydrates, favouring fresh food, such as fruit and vegetables, fish, extra virgin olive oil.

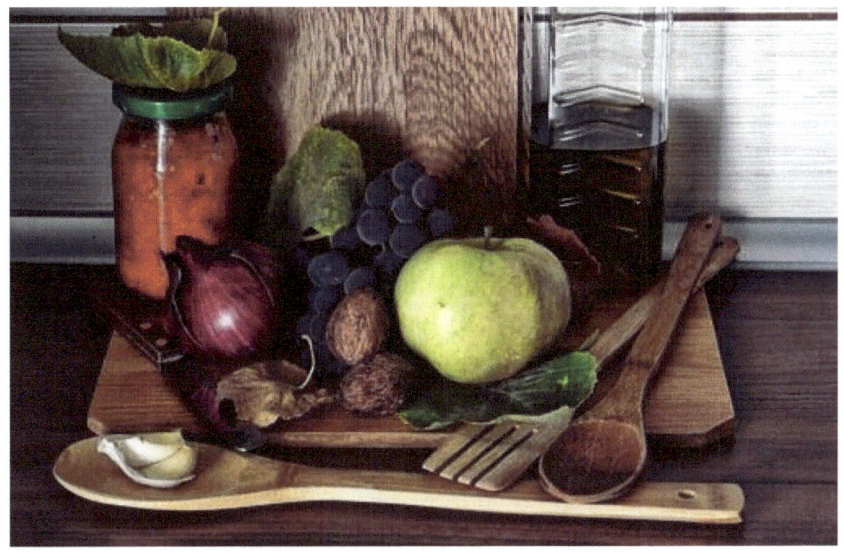

The importance of nutrition

Diet plays a very important role in decreasing the extent and frequency of typical vasomotor disorders of the menopause.

A scientific study published in the American Journal of Clinical Nutrition, conducted in Australia by the University of Queensland, Herston, out of 6040 women in physiological menopause born between 1946 and 1951, observed that women undergoing a rich Mediterranean-style diet fruit and vegetables had a lower risk of suffering from hot flushes and night sweats than those whose diet was high in sugar and fat.

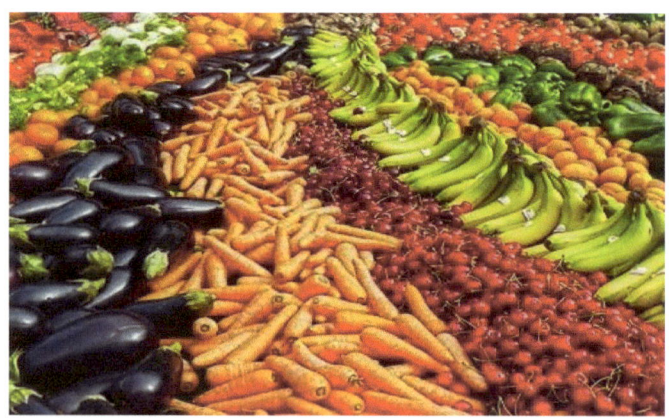

Another study published in Menopause conducted by the Kaiser Permanente Institute, Oakland, California, analyzed 17,473 menopausal women who did not take hormone replacement therapy, in order to establish the effects of a healthy diet with reduced fat intake and increased intake of fruit, vegetables and fibers. The analysis was corrected for age, ethnicity, school level, years since the beginning of menopause, physical activity, presence of depressive symptoms and smoking. From the results it appeared that the women assigned to the group subjected to dietary changes had a reduction of menopausal symptoms until the disappearance, compared to the control group. Although weight loss was not one of the aims of the study, the participants assigned to the dieting group had lost on average 2 kilograms during the study period - a further advantage in the disappearance of vasomotor symptoms in women who had not lost weight.

Other natural remedies

Red clover, cimicifuga racemosa, hypericum, chaste tree, rhubarb root extracts, soy isoflavones, all of them containing phytoestrogens, are just some of the natural products available on the market that are considered useful for counteracting menopausal disorders due to their phytonutrient content.

Proper natural therapy must be able to reduce emotional fluctuations and immediate disturbances related to this transitional period; it should also contain an adequate supply of functional nutrients and should reduce long-term complications of menopause, such as obesity, hypertension, osteoporosis, dyslipidemia, sarcopenia (reduction of the quality and quantity of the muscles); it must always be personalized in terms of dose and combinations of substances (it must be remembered that the effectiveness of these products is not always scientifically proven and some are potentially hepatotoxic).

When buying a natural product you should make sure that it is a titrated and standardized extract, that is a compound in which the active ingredient is really present, effective, in constant measure and content, to be sure of what you are taking (the phytocomplex sometimes needs to be purified from harmful substances present on the plant itself, from pesticides or heavy metals). In Italy, the standardization of the product on the label is at the discretion of the companies that produce the phytotherapics.

Soy is effective in reducing hot flushes, better if taken 2-3 times a day, to control weight gain in menopause and to reduce cholesterol levels; coming largely from the East (the one for human food) is almost all GMO (important to always read the labels of the products you buy and prefer those from organic farming). In the last decade a number of studies have been conducted on the dry extract of soy and the results have been conflicting, in particular on the opportunity to use them in the case of women suffering from hormone-dependent tumours.

Trefoil pratensis is a legume rich in flavonoids, to be associated with soy (as extracts).

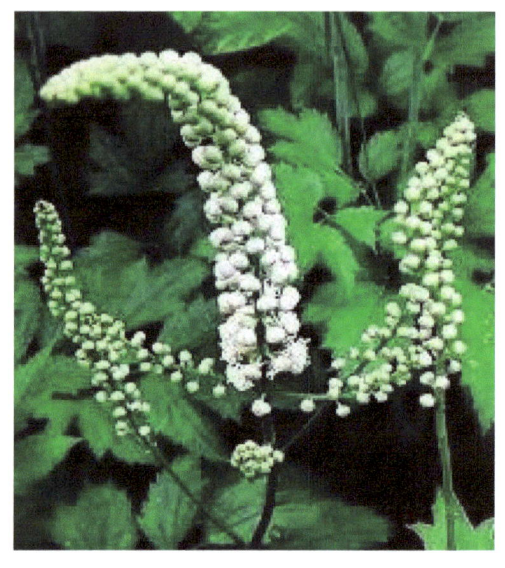

Cimicifuga acts on the central nervous system, on the receptors of serotonin, and for this reason has been used for many years to reduce hot flushes. It is necessary to take it for 3-4 weeks before feeling the benefits and then it should be associated with other products that act in a shorter time. Cimicifuga also reduces night sweats, headache, irritability, palpitations; it exists on the market as a titrated and standardized extract at 2.5%, but contains salicylates, which are not recommended for those suffering from gastritis or are allergic to acetylsalicylic acid.

Oats are available as both grains and flakes, contain betaglucan, which reduces cholesterol levels, and antioxidants and selenium, which help reducing free radicals, protect against cancer (especially the colon) and improve the immune system response. The recommended daily dosage is 3 g per day (contained in 40-50 g of flakes).

Discorea is a climbing herbaceous plant, rich in hormone-like substances, useful for hot flushes, fatigue, vaginal dryness (also for topical use to reduce infections), and according to some studies also to reduce the associated bone loss at menopause. The dry extract is titrated to 20% in diosgenin; the dosage is 400 mg per day to protect bone density and vaginal epithelium.

Some herbal teas could help the mood swings and insomnia, in particular those based on chamomile, lemon balm, mallow, passion flower and hawthorn.

Passiflora incarnata acts as relaxant, improves the quality of sleep so that waking up in the morning is easier and reduces night awakenings.

Hawthorn is useful for those anxious, nervous and inclined to low moods; the menopause by itself turns out to be a stressful event in the long run, and the hawthorn helps to maintain constant values of arterial pressure, reduces anxiety and agitation that precede and follow the hot flushes, improves insomnia resulting in a feeling of relaxation even in the absence of a hypnotic effect; it is available as dry extract or mother tincture (the latter is however on an alcoholic basis).

Melatonin improves the psychic symptoms of menopause and helps to reduce bone loss, but in menopause high doses are indicated and should be taken only on medical advice.

Vitamins and trace elements: essential for metabolism and enzymatic functioning. **Vitamin D** is contained in very few foods so it must be integrated into the diet (according to the Italian Ministry of Health hypovitaminosis is a frequent finding in all age groups), but to avoid poisoning the blood level must first be checked by a normal blood sample . According to the guidelines for osteoporosis, the daily requirement is around 400-800 U/day; exposure to sunlight, in order to provide a proper synthesis of the vitamin, should be done during the hottest hours of the day (from 10 am to about 2 pm) without using sunscreen. Some studies show that a sunscreen SPF15 cream is able to block around 93% of UVB rays.

Vitamins B complex reduce tiredness, irritability, emotional instability, difficulty in concentration and learning often present in menopause, but better not to be taken in the evening for the possible stimulating effects, in particular vitamins **B1** and **B6**.

Vitamin C is useful for improving defences immunity and for the synthesis of collagen (thus to counteract the aging process and vaginal atrophy); to be taken in quantities not exceeding 1 g, better if divided during the day so as not to exceed the capacity of renal filtration.

Lipoic acid or vitamin N reduces bone loss and insulin resistance, has an antioxidant action and activates vitamin E.

Omega-3 act as antioxidants and anti-inflammatories, and are found in some types of algae, seeds and linseed oil, in wild salmon or other fish such as mackerel. Beware of farmed fish as is fed with corn and contains more omega-6, with a pro-inflammatory effect.

Magnesium and Zinc are elements often lacking in menopausal women; however, it is necessary to carry out [a blood test] to measure the dosage in the blood before a possible integration. Among the many beneficial effects of Magnesium, is its stimulation in producing serotonin, while Zinc contributes to the compactness of collagen, and together with calcium and vitamin B6 and has an antioxidant effect. According to the Italian Ministry of Health, the maximum amount of Magnesium contained in the supplements should not exceed 450 mg/day. Magnesium can reduce flushing, more effectively in women who have breast cancer. The easier to tolerate is Magnesium citrate, which has an alkalizing effect, while the other formulas on the market (sulphate, pidolate and chloride) can cause disorders such as diarrhoea, anxiety and insulin resistance.

Red fruits are generally useful (berries, grapes, apples, pomegranates, etc) 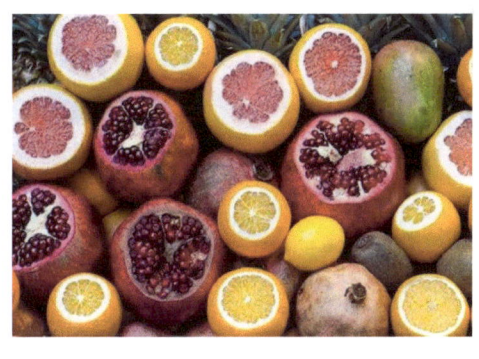 in counteracting the cell aging effects, keeping the muscle tone and the tonicity of sexual organs because are rich in antioxidants, whilst **watermelon** (especially the white part and the skin) helps to preserve the elasticity of the arterial walls.

Pharmacological therapy

To manage the symptoms associated with the climacteric syndrome, especially when they seriously hinder work and social life, appropriate medical treatment tailored to the needs of women, can be used. Namely:

- **hormone replacement therapy (HRT):** it involves the administration of oestrogens alone or in combination with progestogens, using tablets, gels, patches to be applied to the skin or vaginal ring (to be replaced every 3 months), creams or vaginal ovules. Among the mild side effects of hormones are: breast tension, loss or recovery of the menstrual cycle, cramps, abdominal swelling.

- **oral contraceptives:** it is used in the transition phase to regularize the menstrual cycle and alleviate the symptoms of the climacteric.

- **antidepressant drugs:** selective

serotonin reuptake inhibitors (SSRIs) such as paroxetine or venlafaxine and other related; the doses needed to control hot flushes are generally lower than those commonly used to treat depression. Side effects depend on the type of antidepressant and may consist of vertigo, headache, nausea, agitation or drowsiness.

- **Gabapentin**, originally an anti-epileptic drug, nowadays is widely used as a painkiller and has also shown good efficacy against hot flushes.

The indication and/or the need for hormone replacement therapy must be established by the gynaecologist after a careful clinical examination and after a correct evaluation of the risk/benefit ratio for the patient. It has been shown that long-term hormone therapy is associated with an increased risk of breast cancer, gallbladder disease and thromboembolic disorders such as deep vein thrombosis and stroke, so that in women predisposed to such pathological conditions, HRT is contraindicated or (in reality a valid criterion for anyone) the lowest effective hormone dose can be used and for the shortest possible time.

In 2002 the "Women's Health Initiative Study (WHI)" was launched in the USA. Begun in 1991, the study examined 27,347 women aged between 50 and 79 years subjected to hormone replacement therapy. What emerged was a relationship between hormonal substitutive therapy and breast cancer, which led to the interruption of the study after just over 5 years. The increased risk of breast cancer was then confirmed in 2003 by another scientific work conducted in the United Kingdom, the "Million Women Study", which was conducted on over a million women between 50 and 64 years old and was concerned with a certain type of long-term hormone replacement therapy.

Subsequently, further research was carried out, on which basis was established that:
• combined hormone replacement therapy (oestrogens and progesterone) taken after the menopause to alleviate the disorders increases the risk of breast cancer and can

hide its diagnosis. The risk is proportional to the duration of the treatment.
- HRT based on oestrogen alone does not significantly increase the risk of breast cancer, but significantly elevates the risk of endometrial hyperplasia (i.e. of the wall of the uterus) from which endometrial cancer could develop.
- the risk of ovarian cancer may increase depending on the duration of the treatment, although not all epidemiological studies can confirm this possibility.

These risks vary from study to study, depending on the type of hormones administered, the dose and duration of the therapy.

Hormone replacement therapy is also contraindicated in women who had entered the menopause after chemotherapy (especially in case of cancers whose growth is sensitive to oestrogen, such as breast, endometrial and ovarian cancer) or other anticancer treatments.

How I solved the problem of hot flushes

Help in quickly reduce the intensity and frequency of hot flushes and night sweats, which personally experienced about one year after the onset of the symptoms, was given to me by **Acupuncture.**

Acupuncture is the most important therapeutic method in the Traditional Chinese Medicine (TCM). It is a non-pharmacological therapy of exclusively medical competence and scientifically based, which with the insertion of sterile metal needles in selected parts of the human body, promotes the health and the well-being of the individual.

The treatment is almost free of side effects, as was ascertained and recognized by the WHO in 1997.

"Reaching the age of 7 times 7 years, the Ren channel empties, the Chong channel weakens, the tiangui (female cycle) is interrupted, the body begins the decline and the fertility reaches the end"

Huangdi Neijing Suwen, Chapter I (The Emperor's Internal Medicine Canon).

According to Suwen, with the passing of the years the essence of the woman is consumed and her energies are weakened and no longer sufficient to keep the energy channels responsible for fertility open. Although this transformation leads the woman to a new equilibrium, the body is unprepared, leading to the developing of these well-known symptoms.

The millennial Chinese Medicine deals with menopause differently from Western Medicine, seeing it from a fundamentally "energetic" point of view. Eastern medicine is able to see the difficulties that the woman faces when she passes from the procreative phase to the non-fruitful phase of life; these difficulties can originate from an energy imbalance, which is important to restore or to bring on a different axis of balance. In Chinese medicine the hot flushes are caused by an energy imbalance between **yin** and **yang**, which follows the progressive exhaustion of the essence in both its natures.

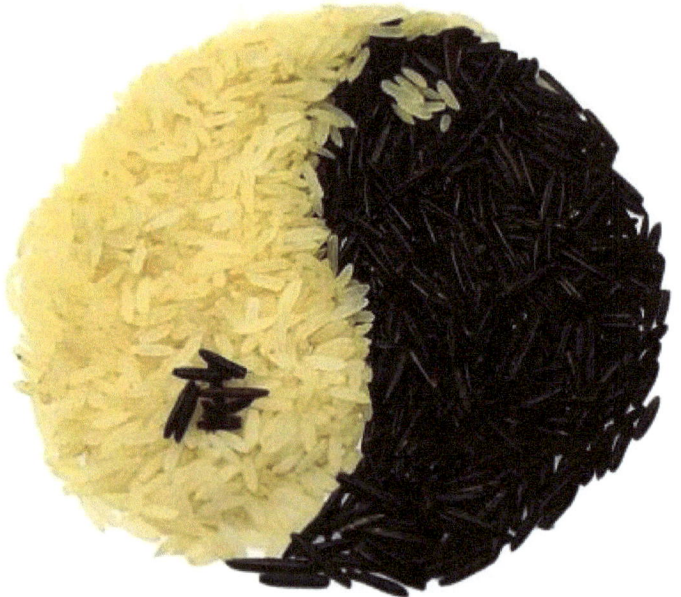

When the yin is deficient, symptoms of heat and dryness will appear, because the body lacks the fluids necessary to lubricate it, causing thirst, hot flushes and constipation. When the yang is insufficient, there will be a lack of heat and abundance of fluids, leading to the development of edema and frequent urination. In daily clinical practice there is often a combination of the two phenomena.

According to the most accredited hypotheses, acupuncture determines a neurophysiological (sensory) stimulation, which acts with different neurobiological mechanisms: a local one, at the points of insertion of the needle, and a central one, on the brain and spinal cord, through the release of useful neurotransmitters to reduce vulnerability to hot flushes, including Serotonin and endorphins, although much of the mechanism of action still remains to be explained.

In addition to this specific effect, it should be added the "placebo effect", which in reality is a neurobiological one, and concerns the patient positive outcome regarding this method. The more positive the expectation, the more beneficial are the effects of acupuncture, which can be amplified by the person's attitude of trust.

Studies have shown that acupuncture increases the oestrogen levels and reduces LH levels; it also increasing the production of endorphin and stabilizing the control of the body temperature. A session every four weeks guarantees a lasting effect of benefits over time.

According to a study published in the journal Menopause by the researchers of the Wake Forest Baptist Medical Center, North Carolina, USA, acupuncture can reduce daily episodes of hot flushes by 37%, both day and night; the first beneficial effects are felt after about eight sessions and are maintained for at least six months after the end of treatment. The research involved 200 menopausal women, aged between 45 and 60, who had on average four episodes a day of hot flushes or night sweats. The study lasted a total of one year and the patients underwent up to a maximum of 20 sessions per head: at the end of the sessions the overall frequency of flushes was reduced by 37% and the benefits were maintained up to six months after the end treatment, with a reduction in incidents that was still around

29%.

A study conducted by a team of Turkish researchers, published on Acupuncture in Medicine of the British Medical Journal group, enrolled a total of 53 women, 27 of which were subjected to acupuncture sessions for 2 months twice a week; the remaining 26 have instead received, without their knowledge, a false treatment based on beveled needles. The results of the test showed that the women in the first group had obtained benefits from acupuncture sessions, with a reduction in hot flushes and mood swings, as a result of the natural increase in oestrogen levels, compared to the second group subjected to fake sessions instead.

A meta-analysis of scientific data performed in 2013 (16 studies, 1155 women) established that acupuncture is effective in treating hot flushes even if its effect is estimated to be inferior to hormone replacement therapy. Another meta-analysis of 2016 (31 studies, 2433 women) shows that acupuncture is associated with a reduction of sleep disorders developed during the menopause and recommends its use for the treatment of symptoms.

Alternative drug therapies, such as acupuncture and physical activity, have proven effective in improving the quality of life of patients with breast cancer; in particular acupuncture and electro acupuncture (a technique that involves the application of small electrical discharges through needles connected to electro stimulators) can integrate traditional therapies to counteract in the most natural way some of the side effects of oncological treatments. The latter method is also being evaluated to alleviate postoperative pain in patients undergoing mastectomy with breast reconstruction.

In general, it can be said that the symptom that responds more quickly to acupuncture is that of <u>hot flushes</u>, while the improvement of <u>sleep disorders</u> often takes more time. To obtain a greater effect in a shorter period of time, it may be indicated to associate a **<u>phytotherapeutic support</u>**.

The use of Chinese herbal medicine in association with acupuncture allows patients to be treated using the full tools of TCM; on the basis of a precise diagnosis it is possible to choose herbs with the most suitable properties to restore the individual energy alteration. Although the setting of herbal therapy is much more complex than a cycle of acupuncture sessions, the advantages offered by this type of treatment should be taken into account, since it is not only limited to reducing vasomotor symptoms and improving quality of sleep, but corrects the basic energy disequilibrium allowing the improvement of many other symptoms.

The use of herbs allows to correct the imbalance created by menopause through small daily treatments, guiding the body towards a harmonious healing process.

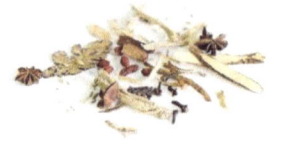 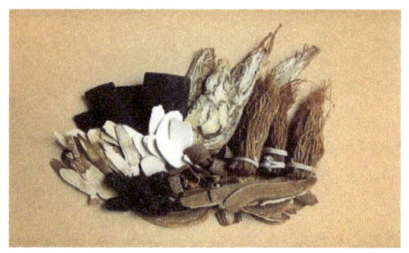

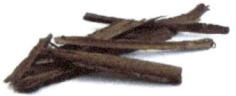

After having drastically reduced the number of episodes of hot flushes and their intensity thanks to acupuncture, the decision of resorting periodically to the consumption of **centrifuged fruit and vegetables** to replace the main meals for short periods of time, especially in place of dinner, has been proved decisive.

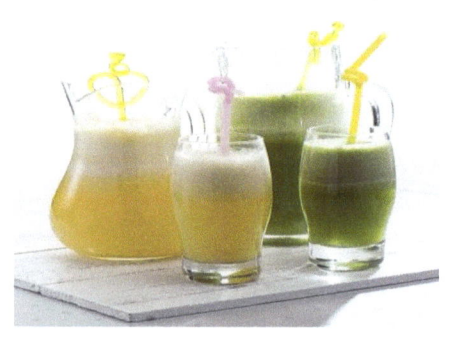

Centrifuged, smoothies and extracts

The **centrifuged** differs from the shake because of the way is prepared: in fact, it is necessary to use a centrifuge, a device able to reduce fruit and vegetables into pulp and then separate the liquid from the fibre, thanks to centrifugal force. In the centrifuged, the peel is not removed and the juice is served raw, keeping in this way all the vitamins, minerals, enzymes and antioxidants present in the selected ingredients. However, in order not to disperse the nutrients, the centrifuged must be drunk immediately.

The centrifuge blades rotate at a very high speed (between 6000 and 18000 rpm) seemingly overheating the products and so reducing their quality. The process also enables air to be incorporated into the liquid, speeding up the oxidation of fruits and vegetables and compromising the nutrients. Compared to a juicer you can extract the juice from other fruit that cannot be squeezed, such as apples, pears, berry, etc. and all kinds of vegetables. The centrifuge is very quick in its task and easy to clean.

In the **smoothie** the pulp of fruits and vegetables, already cleaned, is minced and drunk together with the juice. Also known as "green smoothie", it is definitely denser than the centrifuged thanks to the presence of fibre.

Another difference between centrifuged and smoothies is that, in order to get a glass of centrifuged, you need a much larger quantity of fruit and vegetables, so much so that it would be very difficult eating the equivalent of fruit and vegetables needed to make it. For this reason the centrifuged is definitely more concentrated and nutritious than the smoothie.
Both smoothies and centrifuges can be made with frozen fruits and vegetables, which allow you to taste seasonal products even when they are no longer available on the market. In this case the centrifuged will also contain a lot of water but, given the concentration of nutrients, you will always

have the certainty of assimilating vitamins and minerals in large quantities.

The **extracts** are beverages obtained with a device different from the centrifuge, the extractor, which extracts the juice cold, crushing and sifting the pulp and greatly reducing the waste.

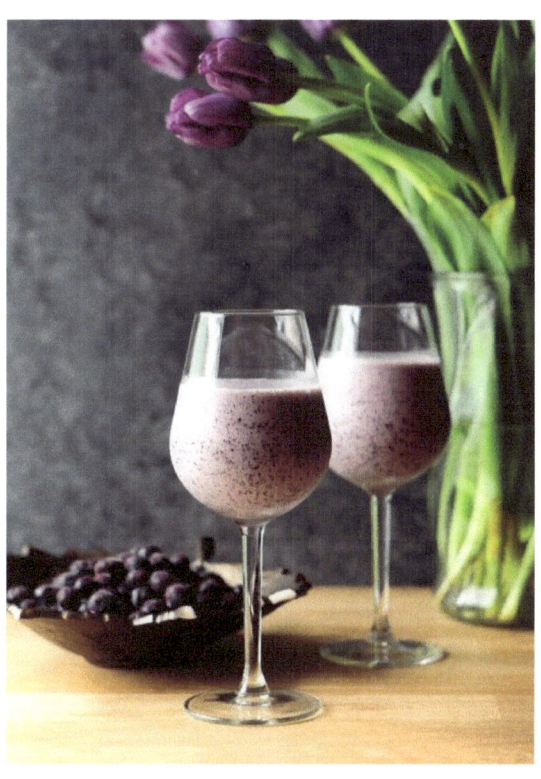

This mechanism of grinding the ingredients is much slower and similar to the movements of chewing, it does not produce heat and thanks to the lower oxidation of the active ingredients used and the greater preservation of the enzymes, the extract is considered a drink of higher quality than the centrifuged. The taste is generally less intense, as nothing remains of the pulp inside the extracted liquid, the appliance takes longer and is more complex to wash and dry. The auger of an extractor must perform a maximum of 60 rpm; the ideal is 30-40 rpm.

Smoothies, fruit shake and juices are considered at a lower level than the extracts and centrifuged; in the manual juicers the plant cell is not dismembered, therefore obtaining a lower enzyme extraction compared to centrifuged and extracted.

As far as long-life bottled juices are concerned, they undergo a pasteurization treatment of at least 70 ° C, which destroys the active elements and the thermolabile vitamins.

Recent scientific studies have shown that drinking fresh juices can help reduce mortality, in addition to promoting the increase of the immune system and weight reduction. It can also promote the prevention of cancer and the detoxification of the organism.
Centrifuged are considered healthy products as they allow to take a mix of fruit and vegetables to drink in one glass, allowing the combination of different types of plant products and creating new and unexpected flavours. Above all, they represent a concentrate of vitamins and nutrients, including several different mineral salts that could hardly been introduced simultaneously, and in such quantities, in our diet.

Globally, a large part of the population - both in the age of development and as adults - do not absorb the quantities of fruit and vegetables recommended by Guidelines and Scientific Societies.

The relationship (inverse association) between scarce consumption of fresh fruit and vegetables, and the risk of developing cancer is listed as "probable" by the World Cancer Research Fund, and it is more evident among smokers and consumers of alcoholic beverages. However, although fruit juices contain phytocompounds, some of which act as antioxidant, minerals, vitamins and in some cases also fibre, the scientific evidence for their role in cancer prevention is still limited, and predominantly confined to the cancer of the pancreas and hepatocellular carcinoma.

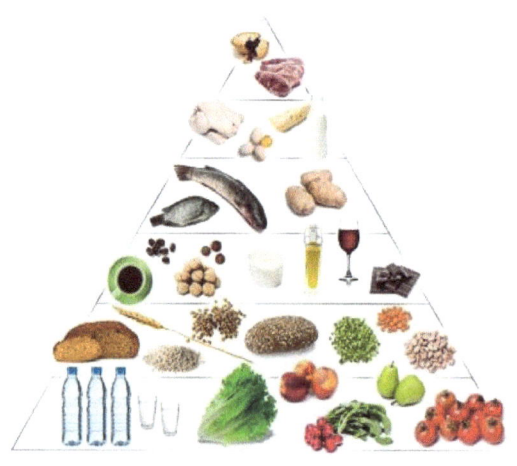

The new food pyramid

How to get optimal fruit and vegetables centrifuged

First of all, you need to get a good quality centrifuge or extractor that allows you to obtain a really nourishing juice; second, a high quantity of fruit and vegetables is required, possibly very fresh, organic and seasonal (because of the greater risk of polluting substances present in the peel); lastly consider the time necessary to wash and clean the fruit, prepare the juice (in particular if using an extractor) and clean up everything later.

Vitamins and other substances contained in the juice extracted from fruit and vegetables are mostly photosensitive and thermolabile, i.e. they are damaged by direct sunlight and heat, so it is recommendable keeping the juice in the refrigerator (in the cold and in the dark), if not consumed immediately. In order to avoid the inactivation of the nutrients when they come into contact with the ambient air, it is possible to keep the juice under vacuum by using special cans and a device that eliminates the air inside. Another method of avoiding oxidation is the addition of antioxidants such as ascorbic acid or Vitamin C (called E300 in the lists of food additives) which slows down the degradation of nutrients; remember to use a teaspoon of wood or ceramic or plastic when you dose antioxidants or with mineral powders in general, as the metal causes the oxidation of a large part of the product in contact with the spoon, while the other materials do not interact with the salts.

To facilitate the absorption of some of the vitamins, such as A, D, E, K (liposoluble), it is useful to add a few drops of a vegetable oil of our liking to our juice (personally I find ginger oil very nice).
Do not use cold fruit and vegetables from the refrigerator and do not consume the juice quickly or too cold to avoid digestive problems. For the same reason, being uncooked and tendentially cold foods, they should be drunk less frequently in the winter months than in the warmer seasons.

Which vegetables:

You can use any type of vegetables according to your tastes, better if combined with spices and fresh roots with additional beneficial properties, such as <u>ginger</u> and <u>turmeric.</u>

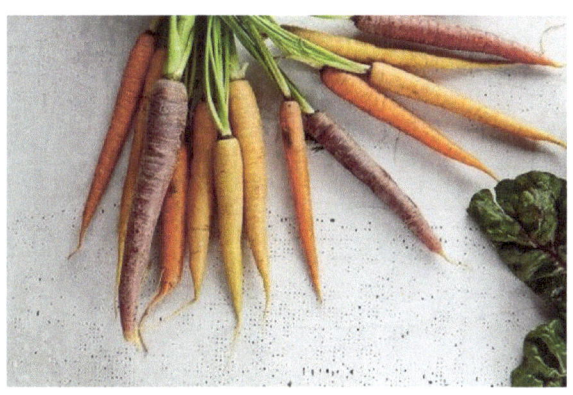

Among the most suitable vegetables is **celery,** which has detoxifying and alkalizing properties, and acts on the reduction of the blood pressure. **Celery** and **cucumber**, which contain few sugars and many nutrients, also produce a lot of juice and give the centrifuged a refreshing and pleasant taste.

Carrots, rich in vitamin A and C and some essential oils, promote digestion, reduce cholesterol levels and counteract the aging process, also the black and purple varieties. Their sweetish taste makes any juice more pleasant to the palate, even in the most daring combinations.

Beetroot has a sweet taste and it is useful in detoxing the liver, kidneys, gallbladder, and its constant intake [can be effective] to counter the disorders of menopause and menstrual pain. Its flavour can be lessened by adding lemon, carrot, ginger and apple.

Fennel has diuretic effects, helps the digestion, prevents muscle cramps and constipation, counteracts aging processes, and strengthens bones and the immune system. It contains many vitamins and minerals, such as calcium, phosphorus and potassium and goes well with apple and lemon juice.

Black cabbage is purifying and possesses many other beneficial properties; add cucumber, mint leaves, apple and lemon juice.

The <u>green leafy vegetables</u> are the richest in chlorophyll (a purifying molecule and chelator also useful for our organism). Vegetables such as **broccoli, spinach**, different varieties of **cabbage, salad, chicory, watercress, spirulina algae**, and bitter herbs like **parsley, coriander, dandelion**, are rich in antioxidant substances and therefore contrast the aging processes; they also are purifying and energizing.

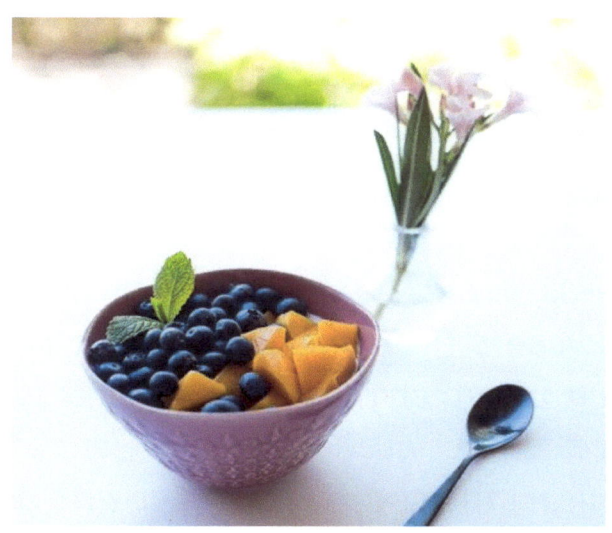

You can combine chard, cabbage, celery, lettuce, cucumber and spinach with a fruit like apple or pear, with the addition of lemon juice.

Which fruits?

Green apples are sourer than the red or the yellow ones, and represent a natural antiseptic, as well as being rich of antioxidants and having alkalizing properties on the organs of our body.

Citrus fruits, such as **lemons** and **limes**, **grapefruits**, **oranges** and **tangerines**, which are rich in vitamins C and group B, strengthen the immune system and combine well with dried fruit, carrots and ginger.
They should always be peeled before being placed in the centrifuge, as their skin is bitter.

Kiwis are also rich in vitamins and trace elements (iron, copper, potassium, vitamin C and E), strengthen the immune system and are thirst-quenching and diuretics. Try pairing them with oranges or with pear, apple and celery for an energizing action.

Fresh **pineapple** combined with fennel is also useful in reducing intestinal meteorism, and together with grapes and all red fruits, helps against cellular aging.

Last tips for a correct consumption

Thanks to their beneficial properties, the juices combining fruit and vegetables are generally suitable for all ages and are especially beneficial in the summer months. However it is advisable consuming them in the right dose, such as one or two glasses a day at most, except in cases of specific liquid diets or particular fasting techniques conducted under medical supervision or other competent personnel. They can integrate a solid diet including whole vegetables and which therefore provides an adequate supply of fibre.

Usually the combination of fruit and vegetables does not presents specific contraindications for the digestive system. However, in some cases, the intake of certain substances such as ginger, for those suffering from gastritis, or sugars (fruit fructose) for those with a tendency to high blood sugar or that suffer from candidiasis (as natural sugars can nourish yeasts and parasites in the body), should be avoided.

In the absence of fibre and of the chewing process, the <u>centrifuged of fruit only</u> can determine glycaemic peaks and an excessive insulin response; therefore it is always recommendable adding at least some carrot, celery or cucumber or, even better, combining half fruit with half vegetables. And obviously, avoid adding sugar if you want a natural and healthy drink.

Juices should not be associated with solid foods, especially proteins and starches, as they cause digestion problems, so it is recommendable drinking them either away from meals, such as about an hour before eating solid food or about two hours after a complete meal, or as a complete replacement of a meal (but always in moderation).

Conclusion:

For a woman facing for the first time the disorders of the menopause, the objective should be trying to create a new, unique and personal psycho-physical balance. Consuming as many natural substances as possible, such as fresh juices and vegetable substances in accordance with the needs of their body, practicing physical activity, as well as meditation and other techniques, such as

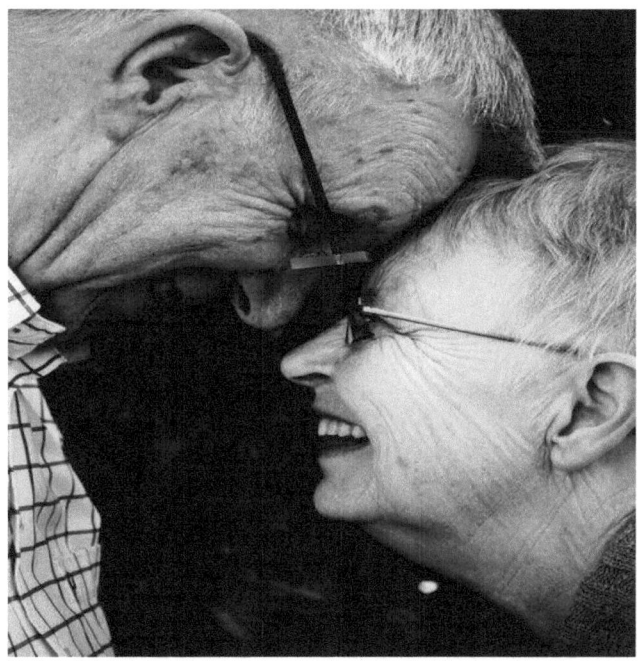

acupuncture, can also help to serenely accept this delicate, albeit natural, transition into a new phase of life, which can still offer many more pleasant surprises and experiences.

BIBLIOGRAPHY

- http://www.my-personaltrainer.it/benessere/climaterio.html

- https://www.alessandragraziottin.it/it/articoli.php/Vampate-non-trascuratele?EW_FATHER=7621&ART_TYPE=AOGGI

- Nancy E. Avis, PhD; Sybil L. Crawford, PhD; Gail Greendale, MD; et al Joyce T. Bromberger, PhD; Susan A. Everson-Rose, PhD, MPH;Ellen B. Gold, PhD; Rachel Hess, MD; Hadine Joffe, MD, MSc; Howard M. Kravitz, DO, MPH; Ping G. Tepper, PhD; Rebecca C. Thurston, PhD, *Duration of Menopausal Vasomotor Symptoms Over the Menopause Transition; for the Study of Women's Health Across the Nation (SWAN), JAMA Intern*

Med. 2015;175(4):531-539. doi:10.1001/jamainternmed.2014.8063

- *http://www.my-personaltrainer.it/salute/vampate-menopausa.html*

- *https://www.nia.nih.gov/health/hot-flushes-what-can-i-do*

- *https://www.nia.nih.gov/health/sleep-problems-and-menopause-what-can-i-do*

- *http://www.vitadidonna.it/news/salute/4698-menopausa-contro-le-vampate-di-calore-perdere-peso-e-una-sana-alimentazione.html*

- *Gloria Richard-Davis, MD1; JoAnn E. Manson, MD, DrPH2, Vasomotor Symptom Duration in Midlife Women—Research Overturns Dogma, JAMA Intern Med. 2015;175(4):540-541. doi:10.1001/jama intern med.2014.8099*

- *https://www.saperesalute.it/vampate-spegnile-cosi*

- *https://www.ilpost.it/2015/12/26/menopausa/*

- Am J Clin Nutr. 2013 May; 97 (5) : 1092-9. doi: 10.3945/ajcn.112.049965. Epub 2013 Apr 3. Fruit, Mediterranean-style, and high-fat and -sugar diets are associated with the risk of night sweats and hot flushes in midlife: results from a prospective cohort study.Herber-Gast GC1, Mishra GD.

- Kroenke, Candyce H.; Caan, Bette J.; Stefanick, Marcia L.; Anderson, Garnet; Brzyski, Robert; Johnson, Karen C.; LeBlanc, Erin; Lee, Cathy; La Croix, Andrea Z.; Park, Hannah Lui; Sims, Stacy T.; Vitolins, Mara; Wallace, Robert. **Effects of a dietary intervention and weight change on**

vasomotor symptoms in the Women's Health Initiative. *Menopause*, 9 July 2012

- Anderson, G., Cummings, S., Freedman, L. S., Furberg, C., Henderson, M., Johnson, S. R., Clark, A. (1998). Design of the Women's Health Initiative clinical trial and observational study. *Controlled Clinical Trials, 19*(1), 61-109.

- www.nhs.uk/Conditions/Sunburn/Pages/Symptoms.asp

- Breast cancer and hormone replacement therapy in the Million Women Study. Million Women Study Collaborators. Lancet 2003; **362**:419-427

- http://www.my-personaltrainer.it/salute/terapia-ormonale-sostitutiva-cancro.html

- www.corsi-ecm-fad.it."Sindrome premestruale e terapie naturali, menopausa e terapie naturali", Dott.ssa Serena Missori.

- Acupuncture for menopausal hot flushes. Dodin S, Blanchet C, Marc I, Ernst E, Wu T, Vaillancourt C, Paquette J, Maunsell E. Cochrane Database Syst Rev. 2013 Jul 30;

- Acupuncture in Menopause (AIM) study: a pragmatic, randomized controlled trial. Avis NE, Coeytaux RR, Isom S, Prevette K, Morgan T. Menopause. 2016 Jun; 23(6):626-37.

- Acupuncture to Reduce Sleep Disturbances in Perimenopausal and Postmenopausal Women: A Systematic Review and Meta-analysis. Chiu HY, Hsieh YJ, Tsai PS. Obstet Gynecol. 2016 Mar; 127 (3):507-15.

- Hormone-replacement therapy: current thinking. Lobo RA. Nat Rev Endocrinol. 2016 Oct 7.

- Singh G.M. et al. Global Burden of Diseases Nutrition and Chronic Diseases Expert Group (NutriCoDE). Global, Regional, and National Consumption of Sugar-Sweetened Beverages, Fruit Juices, and Milk: A Systematic Assessmentof Beverage Intake in 187 Countries. PLoS One (2015) 10(8): e0124845.

- World Cancer Research Fund/American Institute for Cancer Research. Food, Nutrition, Physical Activity, and the

  Prevention of Cancer: a Global Perspective. Washington DC: AICR. 1997.

- Key T.J. Fruit and vegetables and cancer risk. Br J Cancer (2011) 104(1): 6-11.

- Boeing H. et al. Critical review: vegetables and fruit in the prevention of chronic diseases. Eur J Nutr (2012) 51(6): 637-63

- http://wisesociety.it/salute-e-benessere/otto-consigli-per-centrifugati-di-frutta-e-verdura-perfetti/

- http://www.dailyitalia.it/centrifugati-quasi-la-panacea-di-tutti-i-mali/

- http://www.naturalnews.com/045735_juicing_benefits_yeast_overgrowth.html

- https://www.lacucinaitaliana.it/news/salute-e-nutrizione/centrifugati-invernali/

www.ingramcontent.com/pod-product-compliance
Lightning Source LLC
Chambersburg PA
CBHW040227220526
45473CB00001B/157